NCLEX: Genitourinary Disorders

105 Nursing Practice Questions & Rationales to EASILY Crush the NCLEX!

Chase Hassen

Nurse Superhero

© 2015

Disclaimer:

Although the author and publisher have made every effort to ensure that the information in this book was correct at press time, the author and publisher do not assume and hereby disclaim any liability to any party for any loss, damage, or disruption caused by errors or omissions, whether such errors or omissions result from negligence, accident, or any other cause.

This book is not intended as a substitute for the medical advice of physicians. The reader should regularly consult a physician in matters relating to his/her health and particularly with respect to any symptoms that may require diagnosis or medical attention.

All rights reserved. No part of this publication may be reproduced, distributed, or transmitted in any form or by any means, including photocopying, recording, or other electronic or mechanical methods, without the prior written permission of the publisher, except in the case of brief quotations embodied in critical reviews and certain other noncommercial uses permitted by copyright law.

NCLEX®, NCLEX®-RN, and NCLEX®-PN are registered trademarks of the National Council of State Boards of Nursing, Inc. They hold no affiliation with this product.

© Copyright 2015 by Chase Hassen and Nurse Superhero. All rights reserved.

Have you seen my other NCLEX Prep Books?

NCLEX: Respiratory System : 105 Nursing Practice Questions and Rationales to Easily Crush the NCLEX!

NCLEX: Endocrine System : 105 Nursing Practice Questions and Rationales to EASILY Crush the NCLEX!

NCLEX: Cardiovascular System : 105 Nursing Practice and Rationales to Easily Crush the NCLEX!

NCLEX: Emergency Nursing : 105 Practice Questions and Rationales to Easily Crush the NCLEX!

EKG Interpretation: 24 Hours or Less to Easily Pass the ECG Portion of the NCLEX!

Lab Values: 137 Values You Know to Easily Pass The NCLEX!

NCLEX: Genitourinary Disorders

First, I want to give you this FREE gift...

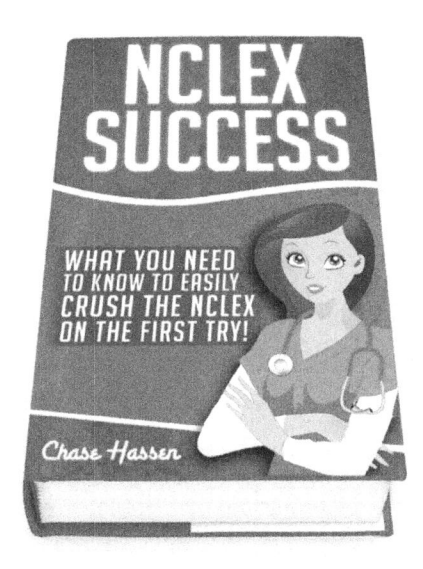

Just to say thanks for downloading my book, I wanted to give you another resource to help you absolutely crush the NCLEX Exam.

For a limited time you can download this book for FREE.

http://bit.ly/1VNGAZ9

NCLEX: Genitourinary Disorders

Table of Contents

First, I want to give you this FREE gift... 4
Chapter 1 : NCLEX: Genitourinary Questions 6
Chapter 2 : NCLEX: Genitourinary Questions, Answers, and Rationales 59
Conclusion 112
Highly Recommended Books for Success 113

Chapter 1 : NCLEX: Genitourinary Questions

The following are 105 questions that will help you study for the NCLEX evaluation. All of the questions are based on things you might need to know in the area of Genitourinary questions. Following the quiz will be the identical questions with the answers and rationales. Compare your answers with the correct ones to see where you may need to study some more. Good luck!

PLEASE NOTE: The answers are located in the next chapter. If you would prefer to see the questions and answers as you review this study guide, visit page 59.

1. You are monitoring a client's urine output, knowing that the average urine output per day in adults is what?
    a. 500 cc
    b. 1000 cc
    c. 1500 cc
    d. 3000 cc

Answer:

NCLEX: Genitourinary Disorders

2. The female client wonders why women have more bladder infections than men. What do you say?
   a. Males drink more water than females.
   b. Women have a shorter urethra than men.
   c. Women have a weaker immune system when compared to men.
   d. Women fail to wipe from back to front when voiding.

Answer:

3. The kidneys regulate the blood pressure by doing what?
   a. Secreting renin into the bloodstream.
   b. Secreting erythropoietin into the bloodstream.
   c. Holding onto more salt in response to an increase in extracellular fluid volume.
   d. Secreting angiotensin II into the bloodstream.

Answer:

4. The client is receiving erythropoietin for what reason?
   a. To increase sodium in the bloodstream, increasing blood pressure.
   b. To stimulate the making of angiotensin II by angiotensin I.
   c. To increase the making of red blood cells by the bone marrow.
   d. To turn off aldosterone production.

Answer:

5. The client has pituitary dysfunction leading to a decrease in production of antidiuretic hormone. What happens to the client's kidneys?
   a. The kidneys cause an increase in blood volume.
   b. Sodium is lost through the kidneys.
   c. Water is lost through the kidneys.
   d. Potassium is lost through the kidneys.

Answer:

6. How do the kidneys respond to acidosis in the bloodstream?
   a. They resorb H+ ions into the bloodstream.
   b. They resorb bicarbonate into the bloodstream.
   c. They hold onto more water.
   d. They excrete bicarbonate into the urine.

Answer:

7. The urinalysis is being evaluated for infection. What amount of organisms indicates the presence of infection?
   a. More than 1000 organisms/cc
   b. More than 10,000 organisms/cc
   c. More than 50,000 organisms/cc
   d. More than 100,000 organisms/cc

Answer:

8. The nurse is instructing a female client on giving a sterile urine specimen. In what order does she give the directions?
   a. Begin the urinary stream.
   b. Separate the labia.
   c. Catch some urine from the urinary stream.
   d. Wipe the meatus from front to back with antiseptic wipes.

Answer:

9. The client is getting a creatinine clearance assessed. What does this measure?
   a. The glomerular filtration rate.
   b. The presence of protein in the urine.
   c. The presence of glucose in the urine.
   d. The volume of urine in 24 hours.

Answer:

10. The client is having a BUN assessed. What does it measure?
    a. The amount of albumin in the urine.
    b. The amount of urea nitrogen in the blood.
    c. The amount of globulin in the blood.
    d. The glomerular filtration rate.

Answer:

11. A normal BUN level is what? (Provide a range).

Answer: _____ mg/dL

12. The BUN level may be artificially increased under what circumstance?
    a. Decreased level of activity
    b. Decreased creatinine levels.
    c. Increased serum protein.
    d. Strenuous activity.

Answer:

13. The most sensitive measure of renal function is what?
    a. BUN level
    b. Creatinine level
    c. Glomerular filtration rate
    d. Uric acid level

Answer:

14. What is true about the sodium level?
    a. It is the major cation in the intracellular space.
    b. Level increases in early kidney failure.
    c. Normal level is 125-135 mEq/L
    d. Level remains constant until end-stage renal failure.

Answer:

15. What is true of the potassium level?
    a. It is the major cation in the extracellular space.
    b. An altered potassium level is the first indicator of renal disease.
    c. A normal level is 5-6 mEq/l
    d. Abnormalities can cause respiratory disease.

Answer:

16. What is true of the phosphorus level?
    a. It carries an inverse relationship between calcium levels.
    b. It can be determined by the thyroid function.
    c. It is the primary mineral in bone.
    d. Levels decrease with renal failure.

Answer:

17. The client is suffering from renal failure. What does renal failure cause with regard to bicarbonate level?
    a. Renal failure raises bicarbonate level.
    b. More bicarbonate is resorbed in renal failure.
    c. Renal failure lowers bicarbonate level.
    d. Renal failure does not affect bicarbonate level.

Answer:

18. The client is suspected of having a renal stone. What is the fastest way to diagnose a kidney stone?
    a. An IVP
    b. A CT scan of the kidney.
    c. A KUB x-ray of the kidneys.
    d. An MRI of the kidneys.

Answer:

NCLEX: Genitourinary Disorders

19. The client is having a KUB x-ray. How do you instruct the client about this procedure?
    a. Have the client be NPO for 8 hours before the procedure.
    b. Tell the client there will be some discomfort with the procedure.
    c. Shield the ovaries from the radiation.
    d. Shield the testicles from the radiation.

Answer:

20. The client is scheduled for an IVP. What do you tell the client?
    a. An IV is not required.
    b. The client does not need to be NPO before the procedure.
    c. Ask the client about allergies to iodine and shellfish.
    d. Restrict fluids before the procedure.

Answer:

21. The client is scheduled for a retrograde pyelogram. How do you instruct the client?
    a. Tell them IV dye will be injected into the veins.
    b. Tell them a cystoscopy will be done after the procedure.
    c. Tell them contrast dye is administered through the urethral catheters.
    d. Tell them to eat a light meal before the procedure.

Answer:

22. After a retrograde pyelogram, nursing interventions include which of the following? Select all that apply.
    a. Assess the client for evidence of sepsis.
    b. Decrease fluid intake after the procedure.
    c. Monitor for ability to void after the procedure.
    d. Monitor for bleeding.
    e. Give IV fluids after the procedure.
    f. Record the client's intake.

Answer:

23. The client is scheduled for a cystography. What do you tell the client?
    a. The client can eat before the procedure.
    b. The client will receive IV contrast.
    c. The client will need a Foley catheter
    d. X-ray pictures are taken when the dye is being inserted into the bladder.

Answer:

24. The client is scheduled for a renal angiogram. How do you instruct the client?
    a. The client will have dye injected via a catheter inserted in the femoral artery.
    b. The client has to be concerned about radioactivity exposure.
    c. The client will have dye injected via a peripheral vein.
    d. CT scan images are taken of the kidneys.

Answer:

25. After a renal angiography, what should the nurse do?
    a. Apply a light sterile dressing to the groin area.
    b. Restrict fluids after the procedure.
    c. Assess the client for reaction to radioactivity.
    d. Assess the client's lower extremity circulation.

Answer:

26. The client is scheduled for a renal ultrasound. What is the advantage of doing a renal ultrasound?
    a. It can assess the renal arteries and veins.
    b. It can be safely given to clients with renal failure.
    c. It is the best way to evaluate a kidney stone.
    d. It uses radioactivity instead of dye to see the kidneys.

Answer:

27. The client is having a CT scan of the kidneys. How do you explain this to the client?
    a. The test uses a magnetic field to assess the structures of the kidneys.
    b. The test can view the organs from many angles.
    c. The test does not require IV contrast.
    d. The client does not need an IV for this procedure.

Answer:

28. The client is scheduled for an MRI of the kidneys. How do you describe this to the client?
    a. It involves the giving of contrast medium.
    b. The client must be fasting for the procedure.
    c. A magnetic field is used to assess the kidney structure.
    d. The client should have an increase in fluids after the procedure.

Answer:

29. The client needs a renal scan. How do you explain this procedure to the client?
    a. You have to ask for allergies to iodine or shellfish
    b. The device involves a scintillator camera to monitor gamma rays
    c. The test does not require an IV
    d. The client should restrict fluids and be fasting before the procedure.

Answer:

30. The client is having a cystoscopy. How do you prepare the client for the procedure?
    a. Tell the client that the bladder and kidneys will be visualized.
    b. Tell the client that an IV contrast will be used.
    c. Tell the client that the exam may be done with or without general anesthesia.
    d. Tell the client to push fluids before the procedure.

Answer:

NCLEX: Genitourinary Disorders

31. Following a cystoscopy under general anesthesia, what nursing intervention is important?
    a. The client can ambulate right after the procedure.
    b. Give prescribed antibiotics one day preprocedure and 3 days postprocedure.
    c. Urine output does not have to be assessed after the procedure.
    d. Expect the urine to be radioactive for 12 hours after the procedure.

Answer:

32. The client is having a cystometrogram. How do you explain this to the client?
    a. The test is a camera test to look inside the bladder.
    b. The test measures the pressure in the bladder.
    c. The client should be fasting before the procedure.
    d. The client should strain while voiding in order to empty out the bladder well.

Answer:

33. During a cystometrogram, the client needs to know the following?
    a. The test will be done under general anesthesia.
    b. IV fluids will fill up the bladder.
    c. The client must indicate when the urge to void is experienced when saline fills the bladder.
    d. The client will not receive any medications during the procedure.

Answer:

34. The client has just had a cystometrogram. What is a post-procedure nursing intervention?
    a. Monitor the client for increased temperature and chills.
    b. Measure the urine output for 24 hours after the procedure.
    c. Tell the client that the urine will be radioactive for 12 hours.
    d. Tell the client to watch for signs of allergy to contrast dye.

Answer:

NCLEX: Genitourinary Disorders

35. The client is having a renal biopsy. What does the client need to know?
    a. The client is placed supine on the bed.
    b. The client will be under general anesthesia.
    c. Surgery is required to expose the kidney.
    d. The client will have a percutaneous sample of the kidney tissue.

Answer:

36. The client is having a renal biopsy. What must be done as part of the procedure?
    a. Hemoglobin, hematocrit and coagulation studies are done before the procedure.
    b. Electrolytes are assessed before the procedure.
    c. The client is placed supine on the operating room table for the procedure.
    d. A light dressing is applied after the procedure is over.

Answer:

37. Following a renal biopsy, what are some nursing interventions?
    a. Help the client ambulate after the procedure.
    b. Monitor the client for signs of hemorrhage.
    c. Monitor the creatinine after the procedure.
    d. Reduce fluids after the procedure to avoid frequent trips to the bathroom.

Answer:

38. The client with urinary retention needs drainage of the bladder. What is the best technique for that?
    a. Push IV fluids to help drain the bladder.
    b. Do a percutaneous bladder tap.
    c. Put in a Foley catheter.
    d. Collect a sterile urine specimen.

Answer:

39. The client has an obstruction of the ureter by a tumor. What is indicated in this situation?
    a. A Foley catheter
    b. A Ureteral catheter
    c. A Percutaneous bladder tap.
    d. A renal biopsy.

Answer:

40. The client is receiving a suprapubic catheter. What is its purpose?
    a. To obtain cells for cytology from the ureters.
    b. To get a renal biopsy.
    c. To drain urine from the bladder.
    d. To drain urine from the renal pelvis.

Answer:

41. The client has a suprapubic catheter. What is a nursing intervention?
    a. Obtain regular serum creatinine.
    b. Avoid kinking the tube to facilitate gravity drainage.
    c. Instill saline into the bladder to flush it out.
    d. Keep the penis clean and dry.

Answer:

42. The client needs a nephrostomy tube. How do you explain this to the client?
    a. The tube is placed through the ureter into the renal pelvis.
    b. The tube is placed into the renal cortex to facilitate excretion.
    c. The tube is placed in the ureter above the site of the blockage.
    d. The tube is placed directly into the kidney to drain urine.

Answer:

NCLEX: Genitourinary Disorders

43. The client is diagnosed with a urinary tract infection. How do you explain this to the client?
    a. The infection is in the bladder only.
    b. The infection is in the kidney only.
    c. The infection is from a hospital-acquired infection.
    d. The infection can be at any part of the urinary tract.

Answer:

44. The most common cause of a nosocomial urinary tract infection is what?
    a. A Foley catheter
    b. Percutaneous renal biopsy
    c. Failing to wipe from front to back
    d. A percutaneous bladder catheter

Answer:

45. The most common organism found in a bladder infection is what?
    a. Candida species
    b. E. coli
    c. Klebsiella pneumoniae
    d. Staph aureus

Answer:

46. The client has acute cystitis. How do you explain this to the client?
    a. It is an infection of the bladder.
    b. It is an infection of the renal pelvis.
    c. It results in hematuria much of the time.
    d. It results in urinary retention.

Answer:

47. A nursing intervention in acute cystitis is what?
    a. Flush the bladder four times daily
    b. Decrease fluid intake to 1000 cc/day
    c. Administer prescribed antibiotics
    d. Place a Foley catheter

Answer:

48. The client has been diagnosed with acute pyelonephritis. How do you explain this to the client?
    a. It is usually the result of blood borne pathogens entering the kidney.
    b. It is usually an ascending infection from the lower urinary tract.
    c. A treatment is to do an IVP.
    d. It is rarely seen in children with vesicoureteral reflux.

Answer:

49. Risk factors for acute pyelonephritis include the following. Select all that apply.
    a. Septic shock
    b. Prostatic hypertrophy
    c. Urinary stones
    d. Increased fluid intake
    e. Being male.
    f. Being pregnant.

Answer:

50. A complication of acute pyelonephritis is what?
    a. Renal stones
    b. Acute cystitis
    c. Septic shock
    d. Dysuria

Answer:

51. Diagnostic tests for acute pyelonephritis include the following:
    a. Urine culture and sensitivities
    b. Percutaneous renal biopsy
    c. Renal stone analysis
    d. IVP

Answer:

52. Nursing interventions for acute pyelonephritis include what?
    a. Placing a Foley catheter
    b. Monitoring intake and output
    c. Providing IV antibiotics
    d. Assisting in an IVP

Answer:

53. The client has urethritis. Common causes of acute urethritis include the following. Select all that apply.
    a. Klebsiella pneumoniae
    b. Chlamydia
    c. E. coli
    d. Trichomonas
    e. Gonorrhea
    f. Pseudomonas

Answer:

54. A common cause of glomerulonephritis includes what?
    a. Systemic lupus erythematosus
    b. Staph infection
    c. Bacteremia
    d. Acute cystitis

Answer:

55. Complications of acute glomerulonephritis include what?
    a. Acute cystitis
    b. Bacteremia
    c. Renal tissue damage
    d. Acute pyelonephritis

Answer:

56. A diagnostic test for glomerulonephritis includes what?
    a. Renal biopsy
    b. Anti-streptococcal antibody test
    c. Urine culture
    d. Urinalysis

Answer:

57. The client has a renal calculus. What is the most common component of urinary tract stones?
   a. Uric acid
   b. Calcium
   c. Bacteria
   d. Phosphate

Answer:

58. A female client has a renal calculus. What is a predisposing factor to having a renal calculus?
   a. Acute pyelonephritis
   b. Acute cystitis
   c. Excess calcium intake
   d. Proteus urinary tract infection

Answer:

59. Common symptoms of a renal calculus include the following:
    a. Colicky abdominal pain
    b. Increased frequency of urination
    c. Pus at the urethral meatus
    d. Fever and chills

Answer:

60. A client has a urinary calculus. What is a nursing intervention?
    a. Tell the client that ultrasound ablation of the stone is likely to happen.
    b. Tell the client that stones are unavoidable.
    c. Give the client the prescribed analgesics.
    d. Tell the client to reduce fluid intake.

Answer:

61. The client requires surgical management of a urinary tract stone. What is an indication for requiring surgery to pass the stone?
   a. A stone that is less than 4 mm in diameter.
   b. The stone is in the bladder.
   c. The stone is associated with severe infection.
   d. The client has normal renal function.

Answer:

62. Nonsurgical ways of removing urinary tract stones include:
   a. Placing a Foley catheter to dilate the urethra
   b. Increase oral fluids
   c. Doing extracorporeal shock wave lithotripsy
   d. Doing a renal biopsy

Answer:

63. Common surgical methods of removing renal calculi include what?
    a. Pyelolithotomy
    b. Ureterolithotomy
    c. Cystotomy
    d. Urethral exposure of stone

Answer:

64. The client has flank pain, hematuria, and back pain following trauma. What has likely happened?
    a. The client has sustained urethral trauma
    b. The client has sustained bladder trauma
    c. The client has sustained liver trauma
    d. The client has sustained renal trauma

Answer:

65. The client has sustained renal trauma. What is a nursing intervention?
   a. Restrict fluids
   b. Provide plasma volume expanders
   c. Measure urine output every shift
   d. Prepare for nephrectomy

Answer:

66. The elderly client is suffering from incontinence. What do you say to help the client?
   a. Tell them this is a normal physiological response to aging.
   b. Tell them that most incontinence is emotionally-based.
   c. Tell them there are medications that can be taken to resolve the symptoms.
   d. Tell them they need surgery to correct the problem.

Answer:

67. The client has sudden urges to void when exposed to running water and must run to the bathroom before spontaneously voiding. What is this called?
    a. Stress incontinence
    b. Urge incontinence
    c. Overflow incontinence
    d. Reflex incontinence

Answer:

68. The client has an inability to void, even with the presence of an urge to void. What is this called?
    a. Urinary retention
    b. Urinary stress incontinence
    c. Urinary urge incontinence
    d. Urinary overflow incontinence

Answer:

69. The client has just had surgery and presents with an over-distended bladder and frequent voiding of small amounts. What is a good nursing response to this condition?
    a. Increase the IV rate.
    b. Put in a Foley catheter
    c. Do a suprapubic bladder catheter
    d. Talk to the doctor about a cystometrogram

Answer:

70. The client has a sudden onset of decreased urine output, proteinuria, fluid retention, decreased serum bicarbonate and increased serum BUN and creatinine. What are some causes? Select all that apply.
    a. Ureteral stone
    b. Acute glomerulonephritis
    c. Hypertension
    d. Fluid overload
    e. BPH
    f. Nephrotoxic drugs

Answer:

NCLEX: Genitourinary Disorders

71. A client has acute renal failure. What is the most severe complication of acute renal failure?
    a. Hyponatremia
    b. Hypernatremia
    c. Hyperkalemia
    d. Hypokalemia

Answer:

72. The client has been diagnosed with chronic renal failure. What is the most common complication of chronic renal failure?
    a. Increased nitrogenous wastes in the blood.
    b. Hyperkalemia
    c. Hyperuricemia
    d. Hypoproteinemia

Answer:

73. Common causes of chronic renal failure include the following. Select all that apply.
    a. Azotemia
    b. Diabetic nephropathy
    c. Hypertension
    d. Cystic kidney disease
    e. Liver failure
    f. Hyperkalemia

Answer:

74. What is the purpose of giving insulin in acute renal failure?
    a. To reduce hyperglycemia.
    b. To put more sodium into the bloodstream.
    c. To facilitate movement of potassium into the cells.
    d. To facilitate the movement of potassium out of the cells.

Answer:

75. The client is undergoing peritoneal dialysis. In what order are the steps given.
    a. Prep the abdomen with providone iodine
    b. Drain fluid out of the peritoneal cavity
    c. Instill 1-2 liters of dialysate into the peritoneal cavity
    d. Allow the dialysate to dwell in the cavity for up to 8 hours.

Answer:

76. The major complication of peritoneal dialysis is what?
    a. Hyperkalemia
    b. Hyponatremia
    c. Renal insufficiency
    d. Peritonitis

Answer:

77. The client is receiving peritoneal dialysis. The dialysate outflow is brown. What does this suggest?
    a. It is from blood cells that have broken down.
    b. There is a possible bowel perforation.
    c. There is a possible bladder perforation.
    d. The dialysis is working and electrolytes are in the dialysate.

Answer:

78. The client has vascular access routes made of grafts for hemodialysis. What is the most common complication?
    a. Hemorrhage from the access site.
    b. Failure of dialysis.
    c. Thrombosis at vascular access route
    d. Septicemia

Answer:

79. What is the major contraindication to getting a renal transplant?
    a. End stage renal disease
    b. Liver disease
    c. Diabetes
    d. Coronary artery disease

Answer:

80. The client is undergoing imminent renal transplant. What must be done prior to the transplant?
    a. Removal of the diseased kidneys.
    b. Withhold dialysis for 24 hours prior to transplant.
    c. Give dialysis within two hours of transplantation.
    d. Give immunosuppressive drugs.

Answer:

81. After a kidney transplant, what is a nursing priority?
    a. Maintain strict adherence to immunosuppressive drugs.
    b. Obtain accurate intake and output measurements
    c. Monitor the color of the urine.
    d. Monitor daily weights and blood pressure readings.

Answer:

82. The client is suffering from hyperacute rejection of a transplanted kidney. What must be done?
    a. Increase immunosuppression drugs
    b. Observe for signs of sepsis
    c. Obtain BUN and creatinine
    d. Remove the transplanted kidney

Answer:

83. The client is suffering from hydronephritis. What is the best test to diagnose this condition?
    a. Renal biopsy
    b. IVP
    c. Excretory urography
    d. Renal function tests

Answer:

84. The client has been identified as having hydronephritis. What is good management for this condition?
    a. Foley catheter placement
    b. Nephrostomy tube placement
    c. Suprapubic bladder tap
    d. Kidney transplant

Answer:

85. The client has been diagnosed with renovascular hypertension. What is a definitive treatment for this condition?
    a. Giving diuretics to lower blood pressure
    b. Eating a low sodium diet
    c. Renal artery bypass
    d. Renal angiography

Answer:

86. What is a complication to the kidneys of surgical ischemia or septic shock?
    a. Chronic renal failure
    b. Urinary obstruction
    c. Tubulointerstitial Nephritis/acute tubular necrosis
    d. Decreased serum potassium

Answer:

87. The nurse is doing teaching on UTIs. What is part of the teaching?
    a. The urinary tract below the urethra is sterile.
    b. Pyelonephritis is an infection of the lower urinary tract.
    c. E. coli is the most common cause of urinary tract infections.
    d. Males get more urinary tract infections than females.

Answer:

88. The normal parts of the urine include the following. Select all that apply.
    a. Protein
    b. Sodium chloride
    c. Ketones
    d. Urea
    e. Epithelial cells
    f. Water

Answer:

89. Children have an increased risk of urinary tract infections. Why is this so?
    a. Decreased immunity to E. coli
    b. Urine is more dilute
    c. Children have a shorter urethra
    d. Children have poor hygiene

Answer:

90. The child has been diagnosed with acute pyelonephritis. What is the most common cause of acute pyelonephritis in children?
    a. Vesicoureteral reflux
    b. Immune deficiency disease
    c. Poor hygiene
    d. A suprapubic urine tap

Answer:

91. A school-aged child has a renal complication of a Strep infection. What is this condition likely to be?
    a. Nephrotic syndrome
    b. Acute pyelonephritis
    c. Acute glomerulonephritis
    d. Strep cystitis

Answer:

92. You are educating a nurse about primary enuresis. What do you say?
    a. The child has had a period of nocturnal dryness before enuresis starts up.
    b. It is more common in boys than in girls.
    c. It is most commonly associated with a urinary tract infection.
    d. The child awakens often during the night.

Answer:

93. The child has been diagnosed with cryptorchidism. What do you tell the parents about this condition?
    a. The testes usually descend when the child is in warm water.
    b. The testicle must be surgically descended in the first year of life.
    c. There is no later risk of testicular cancer if left untreated.
    d. It causes sterility.

Answer:

94. The child has just had surgery for cryptorchidism. What is a priority nursing intervention?
    a. Encourage dietary protein
    b. Assess the cremasteric reflex
    c. Change the diapers frequently
    d. Encourage activity

Answer:

95. A three year old child has diurnal enuresis. Nursing interventions should include what? Select all that apply.
    a. Restrict citrus fruits and high sugar foods
    b. Implement a bedwetting alarm.
    c. Implement a behavior modification star chart.
    d. Restrict dietary fluids.
    e. Encourage a high fiber diet
    f. Administer luteinizing hormone-releasing hormone nasal spray.

Answer:

96. A newborn has been diagnosed with bladder extrophy. What is the purpose of a suprapubic catheter?
    a. It is less painful than bladder catheterization.
    b. It does not require restraining the child like a bladder catheterization would.
    c. It is used to aspirate urine when the child hasn't voided for more than an hour.
    d. It is the only procedure that allows a small catheter to be used on a newborn.

Answer:

97. The nurse checks the clients hourly output of urine as 70 cc/hour. What should the nurse do?
    a. Notify the physician immediately.
    b. Encourage the client to drink extra fluids.
    c. Tell the client to ambulate more.
    d. Recognize that this is a normal urine output.

Answer:

98. What is the purpose of asking the client with pyelonephritis to drink 3000 cc of fluids per day?
    a. To prevent urinary reflux.
    b. To prevent stasis of urine
    c. To decrease urine output
    d. To decrease residual urine

Answer:

99. The nurse is teaching the client about what foods to avoid if the client has calcium oxalate calculi?
    a. Celery
    b. Salmon
    c. Beets
    d. Bacon
    e. Whole wheat bread
    f. Asparagus

Answer:

100. The nurse is teaching a client and family about kidney disease. What does she say?
    a. It takes involvement of 90 percent of nephrons to have acute renal failure.
    b. There is a direct correlation between the amount of urine produced and the severity of kidney disease.
    c. Acute renal failure can happen in the presence of prolonged hypotension.
    d. The best test for kidney failure is the BUN level.

Answer:

101. The nurse is giving a medication to a client with recurrent urinary tract infections. What medication is given?
   a. Levsin
   b. Urecholine
   c. Bactrim DS
   d. Pyridium

Answer:

102. A client is suffering from renal colic due to a ureteral stone. What is a priority nursing intervention?
   a. Straining the urine
   b. Giving morphine sulfate
   c. Monitoring intake and output
   d. Encourage ambulation

Answer:

103. The nurse suspects kidney trauma after an automobile accident. What is a priority that the nurse should report?
a. Lethargy
b. Hypertension
c. Hematuria
d. Bradycardia

Answer:

104. The nurse is caring for a client in acute renal failure. What is the clinical finding that the nurse should monitor as a priority?
a. Infection
b. Pain
c. Oliguria
d. Anemia

Answer:

105. The client has acute renal failure. What lab report indicates the client is uremic?
   a. BUN of 32 mg/dL
   b. Serum calcium of 10.5 mg/d:
   c. Serum potassium of 2.8 mg/dL
   d. Urine specific gravity of 1.030

Answer:

Great Job! On the next chapter, you will see the questions you just answered plus the answers and rationales! I hope you did well!

Chapter 2 : NCLEX: Genitourinary Questions, Answers, and Rationales

The following are the same questions you just took with the answers and rationales. Compare your answers with the correct answers to see where you may need to study further.

1. You are monitoring a client's urine output, knowing that the average urine output per day in adults is what?
   a. 500 cc
   b. 1000 cc
   c. 1500 cc
   d. 3000 cc

Answer: c. The average urine output in an adult is 1500 cc per day.

2. The female client wonders why women have more bladder infections than men. What do you say?
   a. Males drink more water than females.
   b. Women have a shorter urethra than men.
   c. Women have a weaker immune system when compared to men.
   d. Women fail to wipe from back to front when voiding.

Answer: b. Women have a shorter urethra when compared to men so they get bacteria from the stool up into the bladder, causing a bladder infection.

3. The kidneys regulate the blood pressure by doing what?
   a. Secreting renin into the bloodstream.
   b. Secreting erythropoietin into the bloodstream.
   c. Holding onto more salt in response to an increase in extracellular fluid volume.
   d. Secreting angiotensin II into the bloodstream.

Answer: b. The kidneys respond to a decrease in extracellular fluid volume and secrete renin into the bloodstream that transforms into angiotensin I, which is converted to angiotensin II by angiotensin converting enzyme. Angiotensin II causes vasoconstriction which increases blood pressure.

NCLEX: Genitourinary Disorders

4. The client is receiving erythropoietin for what reason?
   a. To increase sodium in the bloodstream, increasing blood pressure.
   b. To stimulate the making of angiotensin II by angiotensin I.
   c. To increase the making of red blood cells by the bone marrow.
   d. To turn off aldosterone production.

Answer: c. Erythropoietin is given to clients in renal failure in order to promote the bone marrow's production of red blood cells.

5. The client has pituitary dysfunction leading to a decrease in production of antidiuretic hormone. What happens to the client's kidneys?
   a. The kidneys cause an increase in blood volume.
   b. Sodium is lost through the kidneys.
   c. Water is lost through the kidneys.
   d. Potassium is lost through the kidneys.

Answer: c. Without antidiuretic hormone, water is lost through the kidneys. ADH is required to resorb water from the kidneys into the bloodstream.

6. How do the kidneys respond to acidosis in the bloodstream?
   a. They resorb H+ ions into the bloodstream.
   b. They resorb bicarbonate into the bloodstream.
   c. They hold onto more water.
   d. They excrete bicarbonate into the urine.

Answer: b. The kidneys respond to acidosis in the bloodstream by resorbing bicarbonate into the bloodstream. The process is not immediate but takes a couple of days.

7. The urinalysis is being evaluated for infection. What amount of organisms indicates the presence of infection?
   a. More than 1000 organisms/cc
   b. More than 10,000 organisms/cc
   c. More than 50,000 organisms/cc
   d. More than 100,000 organisms/cc

Answer: d. A urinalysis with more than 100,000 organisms/cc is indicative of a probable urinary tract infection.

8. The nurse is instructing a female client on giving a sterile urine specimen. In what order does she give the directions?
   a. Begin the urinary stream.
   b. Separate the labia.
   c. Catch some urine from the urinary stream.
   d. Wipe the meatus from front to back with antiseptic wipes.

Answer: b. d. a. c. First the woman separates the labia and then she wipes the meatus from front to back with antiseptic wipes. Begin the urinary stream and then catch some urine from the urinary stream.

9. The client is getting a creatinine clearance assessed. What does this measure?
   a. The glomerular filtration rate.
   b. The presence of protein in the urine.
   c. The presence of glucose in the urine.
   d. The volume of urine in 24 hours.

Answer: a. The creatinine clearance measures the glomerular filtration rate by doing a 24 hour urine collection.

10. The client is having a BUN assessed. What does it measure?
    a. The amount of albumin in the urine.
    b. The amount of urea nitrogen in the blood.
    c. The amount of globulin in the blood.
    d. The glomerular filtration rate.

Answer: b. The BUN measures the amount of urea nitrogen in the blood.

11. A normal BUN level is what? (Provide a range).

Answer: _____10-20_____ mg/dL

12. The BUN level may be artificially increased under what circumstance?
    a. Decreased level of activity
    b. Decreased creatinine levels.
    c. Increased serum protein.
    d. Strenuous activity.

Answer: d. The BUN level may be artificially increased with strenuous activity, GI bleeding, fever, or steroid use.

13. The most sensitive measure of renal function is what?
    a. BUN level
    b. Creatinine level
    c. Glomerular filtration rate
    d. Uric acid level

Answer: c. The most sensitive indicator of renal function is the glomerular filtration rate, followed by the creatinine level. The uric acid level can be a measure of renal function as well.

14. What is true about the sodium level?
    a. It is the major cation in the intracellular space.
    b. Level increases in early kidney failure.
    c. Normal level is 125-135 mEq/L
    d. Level remains constant until end-stage renal failure.

Answer: d. Sodium is the major cation in the extracellular space. The normal level is 135-145 mEq/L. The level remains constant until end-stage renal failure.

15. What is true of the potassium level?
    a. It is the major cation in the extracellular space.
    b. An altered potassium level is the first indicator of renal disease.
    c. A normal level is 5-6 mEq/l
    d. Abnormalities can cause respiratory disease.

Answer: b. An altered potassium level is the first indicator of renal disease. A normal level is 3.5-5 mEq/l. It is the major cation in the intracellular space. Abnormalities can result in cardiac arrhythmias.

16. What is true of the phosphorus level?
    a. It carries an inverse relationship between calcium levels.
    b. It can be determined by the thyroid function.
    c. It is the primary mineral in bone.
    d. Levels decrease with renal failure.

Answer: a. The phosphorus level carries an inverse relationship between the calcium level. It can be determined by the parathyroid glands. Calcium is the major mineral in bone. Levels increase in renal failure.

17. The client is suffering from renal failure. What does renal failure cause with regard to bicarbonate level?
    a. Renal failure raises bicarbonate level.
    b. More bicarbonate is resorbed in renal failure.
    c. Renal failure lowers bicarbonate level.
    d. Renal failure does not affect bicarbonate level.

Answer: c. Renal failure lowers bicarbonate level and causes metabolic acidosis.

18. The client is suspected of having a renal stone. What is the fastest way to diagnose a kidney stone?
    a. An IVP
    b. A CT scan of the kidney.
    c. A KUB x-ray of the kidneys.
    d. An MRI of the kidneys.

Answer: A KUB x-ray stands for "Kidneys, ureters, and bladder" and is the fastest way to detect a kidney stone. An IVP involves the infusion of dye and a CT scan or MRI scan are generally not used to detect a kidney stone.

19. The client is having a KUB x-ray. How do you instruct the client about this procedure?
    a. Have the client be NPO for 8 hours before the procedure.
    b. Tell the client there will be some discomfort with the procedure.
    c. Shield the ovaries from the radiation.
    d. Shield the testicles from the radiation.

Answer: d. During a KUB x-ray, there is no fasting necessary and the procedure causes no pain. The ovaries cannot be shielded because of their location near the kidneys and ureter. The testicles can be shielded, however.

NCLEX: Genitourinary Disorders

20. The client is scheduled for an IVP. What do you tell the client?
    a. An IV is not required.
    b. The client does not need to be NPO before the procedure.
    c. Ask the client about allergies to iodine and shellfish.
    d. Restrict fluids before the procedure.

Answer: c. This is a dye study of the kidneys, ureters and bladder. The client should be NPO for 8 hours before the procedure if possible. An IV is required and the client should be hydrated before the procedure. Ask the client about allergies to iodine and shellfish.

21. The client is scheduled for a retrograde pyelogram. How do you instruct the client?
    a. Tell them IV dye will be injected into the veins.
    b. Tell them a cystoscopy will be done after the procedure.
    c. Tell them contrast dye is administered through the urethral catheters.
    d. Tell them to eat a light meal before the procedure.

Answer: c. Contrast dye will be administered after the cystoscopy through urethral catheters. The client should be NPO after midnight if possible.

22. After a retrograde pyelogram, nursing interventions include which of the following? Select all that apply.
    a. Assess the client for evidence of sepsis.
    b. Decrease fluid intake after the procedure.
    c. Monitor for ability to void after the procedure.
    d. Monitor for bleeding.
    e. Give IV fluids after the procedure.
    f. Record the client's intake.

Answer: a. c. d. After a retrograde pyelogram, the nurse should monitor for evidence of sepsis, increase fluid intake and monitor for ability to void after the procedure. IV fluids are not necessary. Monitor for bleeding. The client's intake does not have to be recorded.

23. The client is scheduled for a cystography. What do you tell the client?
    a. The client can eat before the procedure.
    b. The client will receive IV contrast.
    c. The client will need a Foley catheter
    d. X-ray pictures are taken when the dye is being inserted into the bladder.

Answer: c. The client can have clear liquids for breakfast before the procedure. The dye is inserted via a Foley catheter and x-ray pictures are taken when the dye is being excreted through the urethra.

24. The client is scheduled for a renal angiogram. How do you instruct the client?
    a. The client will have dye injected via a catheter inserted in the femoral artery.
    b. The client has to be concerned about radioactivity exposure.
    c. The client will have dye injected via a peripheral vein.
    d. CT scan images are taken of the kidneys.

Answer: a. The client will have dye injected via a catheter inserted into the femoral artery. There is no radioactivity exposure but the client should be asked about allergies to shellfish or iodine. Regular x-rays are taken of the renal arterial system and a CT scan is not required.

25. After a renal angiography, what should the nurse do?
    a. Apply a light sterile dressing to the groin area.
    b. Restrict fluids after the procedure.
    c. Assess the client for reaction to radioactivity.
    d. Assess the client's lower extremity circulation.

Answer: d. After the procedure, fluids should be increased to facilitate removal of the dye. There is no radioactivity involved. A pressure dressing should be applied to the groin area. Assess the client's lower extremity circulation because occlusion of the femoral artery can occur post-procedure.

26. The client is scheduled for a renal ultrasound. What is the advantage of doing a renal ultrasound?
    a. It can assess the renal arteries and veins.
    b. It can be safely given to clients with renal failure.
    c. It is the best way to evaluate a kidney stone.
    d. It uses radioactivity instead of dye to see the kidneys.

Answer: b. The biggest advantage to doing a renal ultrasound is that it can safely be given to clients with renal failure. It does not use radioactivity or contrast medium.

27. The client is having a CT scan of the kidneys. How do you explain this to the client?
    a. The test uses a magnetic field to assess the structures of the kidneys.
    b. The test can view the organs from many angles.
    c. The test does not require IV contrast.
    d. The client does not need an IV for this procedure.

Answer: b. In a CT scan, the client receives an IV and contrast medium. It can view the kidneys from many different angles. The test uses an x-ray to evaluate the kidneys, not a magnetic field.

28. The client is scheduled for an MRI of the kidneys. How do you describe this to the client?
    a. It involves the giving of contrast medium.
    b. The client must be fasting for the procedure.
    c. A magnetic field is used to assess the kidney structure.
    d. The client should have an increase in fluids after the procedure.

Answer: c. A magnetic field is used to assess the kidney structure. There is no contrast medium and the client does not have to be fasting. There is no need to increase fluids after the procedure.

29. The client needs a renal scan. How do you explain this procedure to the client?
    a. You have to ask for allergies to iodine or shellfish
    b. The device involves a scintillator camera to monitor gamma rays
    c. The test does not require an IV
    d. The client should restrict fluids and be fasting before the procedure.

Answer: b. The renal scan involves a scintillator camera that monitors gamma rays. Radioactive contrast is given by IV. The client does not have to worry about allergies to contrast dye. The client does not have to be fasting and should drink 2-3 glasses of water to be hydrated before the procedure.

NCLEX: Genitourinary Disorders

30. The client is having a cystoscopy. How do you prepare the client for the procedure?
    a. Tell the client that the bladder and kidneys will be visualized.
    b. Tell the client that an IV contrast will be used.
    c. Tell the client that the exam may be done with or without general anesthesia.
    d. Tell the client to push fluids before the procedure.

Answer: c. The cystoscopy may be done with or without general anesthesia. The client should be NPO after midnight if general anesthesia is used. The bladder and ureters are evaluated. It involves a camera but not IV contrast dye.

31. Following a cystoscopy under general anesthesia, what nursing intervention is important?
    a. The client can ambulate right after the procedure.
    b. Give prescribed antibiotics one day preprocedure and 3 days postprocedure.
    c. Urine output does not have to be assessed after the procedure.
    d. Expect the urine to be radioactive for 12 hours after the procedure.

Answer: b. The client should have antibiotics one day preprocedure and 3 days postprocedure. There is no radioactivity involved. The urine output should be assessed for 24 hours because of a risk of urinary retention. The client should be at bedrest after the procedure because of the risk of orthostatic hypotension.

32. The client is having a cystometrogram. How do you explain this to the client?
    a. The test is a camera test to look inside the bladder.
    b. The test measures the pressure in the bladder.
    c. The client should be fasting before the procedure.
    d. The client should strain while voiding in order to empty out the bladder well.

Answer: b. The cystometrogram measures the pressure in the bladder. It does not involve a camera study and the client does not need to be fasting. The client should not strain while voiding or the test will be misinterpreted.

33. During a cystometrogram, the client needs to know the following?
    a. The test will be done under general anesthesia.
    b. IV fluids will fill up the bladder.
    c. The client must indicate when the urge to void is experienced when saline fills the bladder.
    d. The client will not receive any medications during the procedure.

Answer: c. The cystometrogram measures the pressure in the bladder. No IV is necessary. The client must indicate when there is the urge to void when saline is used to fill the bladder. The test is done while the person is awake. The client may receive anticholinergic or cholinergic medication during the procedure.

34. The client has just had a cystometrogram. What is a post-procedure nursing intervention?
    a. Monitor the client for increased temperature and chills.
    b. Measure the urine output for 24 hours after the procedure.
    c. Tell the client that the urine will be radioactive for 12 hours.
    d. Tell the client to watch for signs of allergy to contrast dye.

Answer: a. After the cystometrogram, the nurse must monitor the client for increased temperature, chills, and hematuria. The urine output does not have to be measured after the procedure. There is no radioactivity or dye used in the procedure.

35. The client is having a renal biopsy. What does the client need to know?
    a. The client is placed supine on the bed.
    b. The client will be under general anesthesia.
    c. Surgery is required to expose the kidney.
    d. The client will have a percutaneous sample of the kidney tissue.

Answer: d. The client will have a percutaneous sample of the kidney tissue under local anesthesia. No surgery is required. The client is placed prone with a pillow under the abdomen.

NCLEX: Genitourinary Disorders

36. The client is having a renal biopsy. What must be done as part of the procedure?
    a. Hemoglobin, hematocrit and coagulation studies are done before the procedure.
    b. Electrolytes are assessed before the procedure.
    c. The client is placed supine on the operating room table for the procedure.
    d. A light dressing is applied after the procedure is over.

Answer: a. A hemoglobin, hematocrit, and coagulation studies are done before the procedure. Electrolytes are not necessary. The client is placed prone on the table with a pillow under the abdomen. Pressure is applied to the site for twenty minutes after the procedure.

37. Following a renal biopsy, what are some nursing interventions?
    a. Help the client ambulate after the procedure.
    b. Monitor the client for signs of hemorrhage.
    c. Monitor the creatinine after the procedure.
    d. Reduce fluids after the procedure to avoid frequent trips to the bathroom.

Answer: b. The client should be flat in bed for 24 hours after the procedure. Monitor the client for signs of hemorrhage postprocedure. A postprocedure creatinine does not have to be assessed. Fluids should be increased after the procedure.

38. The client with urinary retention needs drainage of the bladder. What is the best technique for that?
   a. Push IV fluids to help drain the bladder.
   b. Do a percutaneous bladder tap.
   c. Put in a Foley catheter.
   d. Collect a sterile urine specimen.

Answer: c. A Foley catheter can effectively drain the bladder without the need for a percutaneous bladder tap. A sterile specimen can be gotten from the Foley catheter once it is inserted.

39. The client has an obstruction of the ureter by a tumor. What is indicated in this situation?
   a. A Foley catheter
   b. A Ureteral catheter
   c. A Percutaneous bladder tap.
   d. A renal biopsy.

Answer: b. A ureteral catheter can bypass the tumor and drain the kidney. A Foley catheter or a percutaneous bladder tap will not help. A renal biopsy is not indicated.

40. The client is receiving a suprapubic catheter. What is its purpose?
    a. To obtain cells for cytology from the ureters.
    b. To get a renal biopsy.
    c. To drain urine from the bladder.
    d. To drain urine from the renal pelvis.

Answer: c. The purpose of a suprapubic catheter is to drain urine from the bladder.

41. The client has a suprapubic catheter. What is a nursing intervention?
    a. Obtain regular serum creatinine.
    b. Avoid kinking the tube to facilitate gravity drainage.
    c. Instill saline into the bladder to flush it out.
    d. Keep the penis clean and dry.

Answer: b. The suprapubic catheter is prone to kinking and poor drainage so it must be avoided. A serum creatinine does not need to be ordered. Saline is not instilled into the bladder unless there is blockage. The penis is not involved in a suprapubic catheter.

42. The client needs a nephrostomy tube. How do you explain this to the client?
    a. The tube is placed through the ureter into the renal pelvis.
    b. The tube is placed into the renal cortex to facilitate excretion.
    c. The tube is placed in the ureter above the site of the blockage.
    d. The tube is placed directly into the kidney to drain urine.

Answer: d. In a nephrostomy tube, the tube is placed directly into the kidney in order to drain urine from the kidney.

43. The client is diagnosed with a urinary tract infection. How do you explain this to the client?
    a. The infection is in the bladder only.
    b. The infection is in the kidney only.
    c. The infection is from a hospital-acquired infection.
    d. The infection can be at any part of the urinary tract.

Answer: d. A UTI can involve any part of the urinary tract and can be community-acquired or hospital-acquired.

44. The most common cause of a nosocomial urinary tract infection is what?
    a. A Foley catheter
    b. Percutaneous renal biopsy
    c. Failing to wipe from front to back
    d. A percutaneous bladder catheter

Answer: a. The most common cause of a nosocomial urinary tract infection is a urinary catheter, such as a Foley catheter.

45. The most common organism found in a bladder infection is what?
    a. Candida species
    b. E. coli
    c. Klebsiella pneumoniae
    d. Staph aureus

Answer: b. The most common organism found in a bladder infection is E. coli.

46. The client has acute cystitis. How do you explain this to the client?
    a. It is an infection of the bladder.
    b. It is an infection of the renal pelvis.
    c. It results in hematuria much of the time.
    d. It results in urinary retention.

Answer: a. The client with cystitis has an infection of the bladder. It does not involve the kidneys and hematuria is present only some of the time. It does not result in urinary retention but rather urinary frequency and urgency.

47. A nursing intervention in acute cystitis is what?
    a. Flush the bladder four times daily
    b. Decrease fluid intake to 1000 cc/day
    c. Administer prescribed antibiotics
    d. Place a Foley catheter

Answer: c. A nursing intervention is to administer prescribed antibiotics. Fluid intake should be increased to up to 3000 cc/day. The bladder does not have to be flushed and a Foley catheter does not have to be placed.

48. The client has been diagnosed with acute pyelonephritis. How do you explain this to the client?
    a. It is usually the result of blood borne pathogens entering the kidney.
    b. It is usually an ascending infection from the lower urinary tract.
    c. A treatment is to do an IVP.
    d. It is rarely seen in children with vesicoureteral reflux.

Answer: b. Acute pyelonephritis is a kidney infection usually caused by an ascending infection from the lower urinary tract. It is treated with antibiotics. It is common in children with vesicoureteral reflux.

49. Risk factors for acute pyelonephritis include the following. Select all that apply.
    a. Septic shock
    b. Prostatic hypertrophy
    c. Urinary stones
    d. Increased fluid intake
    e. Being male.
    f. Being pregnant.

Answer: b. c. f. Risk factors for acute pyelonephritis include prostatic hypertrophy, urinary stones and being pregnant. Being male is not a risk factor nor is increased fluid intake. Septic shock is a complication of acute pyelonephritis.

50. A complication of acute pyelonephritis is what?
    a. Renal stones
    b. Acute cystitis
    c. Septic shock
    d. Dysuria

Answer: c. A complication of acute pyelonephritis is septic shock. Acute cystitis and renal stones are risk factors for acute pyelonephritis and dysuria is a symptom of the condition.

51. Diagnostic tests for acute pyelonephritis include the following:
    a. Urine culture and sensitivities
    b. Percutaneous renal biopsy
    c. Renal stone analysis
    d. IVP

Answer: a. A diagnostic test for acute pyelonephritis is a urine culture and sensitivities. A renal biopsy and renal stone analysis are not necessary. An IVP would not be helpful in diagnosing acute pyelonephritis.

52. Nursing interventions for acute pyelonephritis include what?
    a. Placing a Foley catheter
    b. Monitoring intake and output
    c. Providing IV antibiotics
    d. Assisting in an IVP

Answer: c. A nursing intervention for the management of acute pyelonephritis includes providing IV antibiotics initially, followed by oral antibiotics. A Foley catheter is not necessary nor is measuring the intake and output. An IVP is not necessary.

53. The client has urethritis. Common causes of acute urethritis include the following. Select all that apply.
    a. Klebsiella pneumoniae
    b. Chlamydia
    c. E. coli
    d. Trichomonas
    e. Gonorrhea
    f. Pseudomonas

Answer: b. d. e. Common causes of acute urethritis include Chlamydia, Trichomonas, and gonorrhea.

54. A common cause of glomerulonephritis includes what?
    a. Systemic lupus erythematosus
    b. Staph infection
    c. Bacteremia
    d. Acute cystitis

Answer: a. A common cause of acute glomerulonephritis is an autoimmune disease like systemic lupus erythematosus or scleroderma. A streptococcal infection can cause glomerulonephritis as well. It is not the result of a staph infection, bacteremia, or acute cystitis.

55. Complications of acute glomerulonephritis include what?
    a. Acute cystitis
    b. Bacteremia
    c. Renal tissue damage
    d. Acute pyelonephritis

Answer: c. A complication of acute glomerulonephritis includes renal tissue damage. The other choices are not complications of acute glomerulonephritis.

56. A diagnostic test for glomerulonephritis includes what?
    a. Renal biopsy
    b. Anti-streptococcal antibody test
    c. Urine culture
    d. Urinalysis

Answer: a. A good diagnostic test is a renal biopsy looking for antiglomerular-basement membrane antibodies. An anti-streptococcal antibody test, urinalysis or urine culture will not help diagnose glomerulonephritis.

57. The client has a renal calculus. What is the most common component of urinary tract stones?
    a. Uric acid
    b. Calcium
    c. Bacteria
    d. Phosphate

Answer: b. The most common component of a urinary tract stone is calcium. Uric acid accounts for less than 5 percent of all renal calculi.

58. A female client has a renal calculus. What is a predisposing factor to having a renal calculus?
    a. Acute pyelonephritis
    b. Acute cystitis
    c. Excess calcium intake
    d. Proteus urinary tract infection

Answer: d. A predisposing factor to developing a renal calculus in women is a Proteus urinary tract infection.

59. Common symptoms of a renal calculus include the following:
    a. Colicky abdominal pain
    b. Increased frequency of urination
    c. Pus at the urethral meatus
    d. Fever and chills

Answer: a. A common symptom of a renal calculus is colicky abdominal pain when the calculus travels to the ureter. Increased frequency of urination, pus at the urethral meatus and fever/chills are not signs of a renal calculus.

60. A client has a urinary calculus. What is a nursing intervention?
    a. Tell the client that ultrasound ablation of the stone is likely to happen.
    b. Tell the client that stones are unavoidable.
    c. Give the client the prescribed analgesics.
    d. Tell the client to reduce fluid intake.

Answer: c. The nurse should give the prescribed analgesics and should reassure the client that most stones are small enough to pass. The client should be taught ways to prevent stones and should be encouraged to increase fluid intake.

61. The client requires surgical management of a urinary tract stone. What is an indication for requiring surgery to pass the stone?
    a. A stone that is less than 4 mm in diameter.
    b. The stone is in the bladder.
    c. The stone is associated with severe infection.
    d. The client has normal renal function.

Answer: c. The stone should be removed if it doesn't pass spontaneously out of the ureter or if it is associated with bacteriuria or severe infection. It should also be removed if it is adversely affecting renal function.

62. Nonsurgical ways of removing urinary tract stones include:
    a. Placing a Foley catheter to dilate the urethra
    b. Increase oral fluids
    c. Doing extracorporeal shock wave lithotripsy
    d. Doing a renal biopsy

Answer: c. Extracorporeal shock wave lithotripsy can break up a stone into smaller pieces so they can be passed separately.

63. Common surgical methods of removing renal calculi include what?
    a. Pyelolithotomy
    b. Ureterolithotomy
    c. Cystotomy
    d. Urethral exposure of stone

Answer: a. If the client has a renal calculus, the incision must be done into the renal pelvis to remove the stone. This involves doing a pyelolithotomy.

64. The client has flank pain, hematuria, and back pain following trauma. What has likely happened?
    a. The client has sustained urethral trauma
    b. The client has sustained bladder trauma
    c. The client has sustained liver trauma
    d. The client has sustained renal trauma

Answer: d. The client has symptoms of flank pain, hematuria and back pain most likely indicating renal trauma.

65. The client has sustained renal trauma. What is a nursing intervention?
    a. Restrict fluids
    b. Provide plasma volume expanders
    c. Measure urine output every shift
    d. Prepare for nephrectomy

Answer: b. In a renal trauma situation, the nurse must give extra fluids, provide plasma volume expanders, and measure urine output every hour. A nephrectomy is not always necessary as the kidney may heal itself.

66. The elderly client is suffering from incontinence. What do you say to help the client?
   a. Tell them this is a normal physiological response to aging.
   b. Tell them that most incontinence is emotionally-based.
   c. Tell them there are medications that can be taken to resolve the symptoms.
   d. Tell them they need surgery to correct the problem.

Answer: c. Incontinence is not a normal physiological response to aging. There are medications that can help resolve the symptoms. Incontinence is not an emotional problem and surgery is not often recommended.

67. The client has sudden urges to void when exposed to running water and must run to the bathroom before spontaneously voiding. What is this called?
   a. Stress incontinence
   b. Urge incontinence
   c. Overflow incontinence
   d. Reflex incontinence

Answer: b. The symptoms are most suggestive of urge incontinence.

68. The client has an inability to void, even with the presence of an urge to void. What is this called?
   a. Urinary retention
   b. Urinary stress incontinence
   c. Urinary urge incontinence
   d. Urinary overflow incontinence

Answer: a. The inability to void, even with the presence of an urge to void is called urinary retention.

69. The client has just had surgery and presents with an over-distended bladder and frequent voiding of small amounts. What is a good nursing response to this condition?
   a. Increase the IV rate.
   b. Put in a Foley catheter
   c. Do a suprapubic bladder catheter
   d. Talk to the doctor about a cystometrogram

Answer: b. The client likely has post-operative urinary retention which can be relieved by inserting a Foley catheter until the problem is resolved. A suprapubic bladder catheter and cystometrogram are unnecessary.

70. The client has a sudden onset of decreased urine output, proteinuria, fluid retention, decreased serum bicarbonate and increased serum BUN and creatinine. What are some causes? Select all that apply.
    a. Ureteral stone
    b. Acute glomerulonephritis
    c. Hypertension
    d. Fluid overload
    e. BPH
    f. Nephrotoxic drugs

Answer: b. e. f. Common causes of these symptoms of acute renal failure include acute glomerulonephritis, BPH and nephrotoxic drugs. Other causes are cancer of the prostate or kidneys.

71. A client has acute renal failure. What is the most severe complication of acute renal failure?
    a. Hyponatremia
    b. Hypernatremia
    c. Hyperkalemia
    d. Hypokalemia

Answer: c. The most serious complication of acute renal failure is hyperkalemia.

72. The client has been diagnosed with chronic renal failure. What is the most common complication of chronic renal failure?
    a. Increased nitrogenous wastes in the blood.
    b. Hyperkalemia
    c. Hyperuricemia
    d. Hypoproteinemia

Answer: a. The most common complication of chronic renal failure is increased nitrogenous wastes in the bloodstream.

73. Common causes of chronic renal failure include the following. Select all that apply.
    a. Azotemia
    b. Diabetic nephropathy
    c. Hypertension
    d. Cystic kidney disease
    e. Liver failure
    f. Hyperkalemia

Answer: b. c. d. Common causes of chronic renal failure include diabetic nephropathy, hypertension, glomerulonephritis and cystic kidney disease. Azotemia is a complication of chronic renal failure and hyperkalemia is a complication of acute renal failure.

74. What is the purpose of giving insulin in acute renal failure?
    a. To reduce hyperglycemia.
    b. To put more sodium into the bloodstream.
    c. To facilitate movement of potassium into the cells.
    d. To facilitate the movement of potassium out of the cells.

Answer: c. The purpose of giving insulin in acute renal failure is to facilitate movement of potassium into the cells. IV glucose is given to prevent hypoglycemia.

75. The client is undergoing peritoneal dialysis. In what order are the steps given.
    a. Prep the abdomen with providone iodine
    b. Drain fluid out of the peritoneal cavity
    c. Instill 1-2 liters of dialysate into the peritoneal cavity
    d. Allow the dialysate to dwell in the cavity for up to 8 hours.

Answer: a. c. d. b. First the abdomen is prepped and then the dialysate is instilled into the peritoneal cavity. It is allowed to dwell in the cavity for 30 minutes to 8 hours and then is drained out of the peritoneal cavity.

76. The major complication of peritoneal dialysis is what?
    a. Hyperkalemia
    b. Hyponatremia
    c. Renal insufficiency
    d. Peritonitis

Answer: d. The major complication of peritoneal dialysis is peritonitis from contamination of the dialysate.

77. The client is receiving peritoneal dialysis. The dialysate outflow is brown. What does this suggest?
    a. It is from blood cells that have broken down.
    b. There is a possible bowel perforation.
    c. There is a possible bladder perforation.
    d. The dialysis is working and electrolytes are in the dialysate.

Answer: b. Brown outflow indicates the possibility of a bowel perforation. Yellow outflow indicates a possible bladder perforation.

78. The client has vascular access routes made of grafts for hemodialysis. What is the most common complication?
   a. Hemorrhage from the access site.
   b. Failure of dialysis.
   c. Thrombosis at vascular access route
   d. Septicemia

Answer: c. The most common complication of vascular access routes for hemodialysis is thrombosis at the graft site.

79. What is the major contraindication to getting a renal transplant?
   a. End stage renal disease
   b. Liver disease
   c. Diabetes
   d. Coronary artery disease

Answer: d. The major contraindication to getting a renal transplant is having coronary artery disease.

80. The client is undergoing imminent renal transplant. What must be done prior to the transplant?
   a. Removal of the diseased kidneys.
   b. Withhold dialysis for 24 hours prior to transplant.
   c. Give dialysis within two hours of transplantation.
   d. Give immunosuppressive drugs.

Answer: c. Prior to transplantation, the client must have dialysis within 2 hours of the procedure. Immunosuppressant drugs are given after the transplant and the diseased kidneys are not removed.

81. After a kidney transplant, what is a nursing priority?
   a. Maintain strict adherence to immunosuppressive drugs.
   b. Obtain accurate intake and output measurements
   c. Monitor the color of the urine.
   d. Monitor daily weights and blood pressure readings.

Answer: a. While all things must be done, the priority nursing intervention is to maintain strict adherence to immunosuppressive drugs to prevent transplant rejection.

82. The client is suffering from hyperacute rejection of a transplanted kidney. What must be done?
    a. Increase immunosuppression drugs
    b. Observe for signs of sepsis
    c. Obtain BUN and creatinine
    d. Remove the transplanted kidney

Answer: d. If the client is suffering from hyperacute rejection of a transplanted kidney (within 48 hours of transplant), the transplanted kidney must be removed. If the rejection is just "acute", immunosuppressive drugs may make a difference.

83. The client is suffering from hydronephritis. What is the best test to diagnose this condition?
    a. Renal biopsy
    b. IVP
    c. Excretory urography
    d. Renal function tests

Answer: c. Hydronephritis is a condition where the kidney pelvis dilates and there is backup of urine into the kidney. The best test to diagnose this condition is an excretory urography evaluation. Renal function tests are not specific enough and a renal biopsy is not indicated. An IVP is not indicated.

84. The client has been identified as having hydronephritis. What is good management for this condition?
   a. Foley catheter placement
   b. Nephrostomy tube placement
   c. Suprapubic bladder tap
   d. Kidney transplant

Answer: b. The best treatment for hydronephritis is the placement of a nephrostomy tube to facilitate drainage from the kidney. A Foley catheter and Suprapubic bladder tap will not help and a kidney transplant is not indicated.

85. The client has been diagnosed with renovascular hypertension. What is a definitive treatment for this condition?
   a. Giving diuretics to lower blood pressure
   b. Eating a low sodium diet
   c. Renal artery bypass
   d. Renal angiography

Answer: c. The definitive treatment for renovascular hypertension is a renal artery bypass. Diuretics and a low sodium diet are just temporary measures and a renal angiography is used to diagnose the disease.

86. What is a complication to the kidneys of surgical ischemia or septic shock?
a. Chronic renal failure
b. Urinary obstruction
c. Tubulointerstitial Nephritis/acute tubular necrosis
d. Decreased serum potassium

Answer: c. A complication of renal trauma, surgical ischemia, or septic shock is acute tubular necrosis or tubulointerstitial nephritis. There is acute renal failure with elevation of the serum potassium.

87. The nurse is doing teaching on UTIs. What is part of the teaching?
a. The urinary tract below the urethra is sterile.
b. Pyelonephritis is an infection of the lower urinary tract.
c. E. coli is the most common cause of urinary tract infections.
d. Males get more urinary tract infections than females.

Answer: c. E. coli is the most common cause of UTIs. Females are more prone to getting UTIs than males and the area below the urethra is not sterile. Pyelonephritis is an infection of the upper urinary tract.

88. The normal parts of the urine include the following. Select all that apply.
    a. Protein
    b. Sodium chloride
    c. Ketones
    d. Urea
    e. Epithelial cells
    f. Water

Answer: b. d. f. Urine consists of water, urea and sodium chloride. Protein in the urine is a problem in renal failure and ketones come from diabetic ketoacidosis. Epithelial cells usually come from an incorrectly obtained urine specimen.

89. Children have an increased risk of urinary tract infections. Why is this so?
    a. Decreased immunity to E. coli
    b. Urine is more dilute
    c. Children have a shorter urethra
    d. Children have poor hygiene

Answer: c. Children have an increased risk of urinary tract infections because they have shorter urethras.

90. The child has been diagnosed with acute pyelonephritis. What is the most common cause of acute pyelonephritis in children?
   a. Vesicoureteral reflux
   b. Immune deficiency disease
   c. Poor hygiene
   d. A suprapubic urine tap

Answer: a. The most common cause of acute pyelonephritis in children is vesicoureteral reflux, which can be congenital.

91. A school-aged child has a renal complication of a Strep infection. What is this condition likely to be?
   a. Nephrotic syndrome
   b. Acute pyelonephritis
   c. Acute glomerulonephritis
   d. Strep cystitis

Answer: c. A renal complication of a strep infection is acute glomerulonephritis.

92. You are educating a nurse about primary enuresis. What do you say?
    a. The child has had a period of nocturnal dryness before enuresis starts up.
    b. It is more common in boys than in girls.
    c. It is most commonly associated with a urinary tract infection.
    d. The child awakens often during the night.

Answer: b. Primary enuresis most often occurs in boys. They never have a period of dryness at night. It is not usually associated with a urinary tract infection. The child rarely awakens at night.

93. The child has been diagnosed with cryptorchidism. What do you tell the parents about this condition?
    a. The testes usually descend when the child is in warm water.
    b. The testicle must be surgically descended in the first year of life.
    c. There is no later risk of testicular cancer if left untreated.
    d. It causes sterility.

Answer: b. An undescended testicle must be surgically managed in the first year of life to avoid the risk of later having testicular cancer. If just one testicle is affected, the child is still fertile. An undescended testicle will not descend when the child is in warm water.

94. The child has just had surgery for cryptorchidism. What is a priority nursing intervention?
    a. Encourage dietary protein
    b. Assess the cremasteric reflex
    c. Change the diapers frequently
    d. Encourage activity

Answer: c. After surgery, the diaper should be changed frequently in order to prevent infection.

95. A three year old child has diurnal enuresis. Nursing interventions should include what? Select all that apply.
    a. Restrict citrus fruits and high sugar foods
    b. Implement a bedwetting alarm.
    c. Implement a behavior modification star chart.
    d. Restrict dietary fluids.
    e. Encourage a high fiber diet
    f. Administer luteinizing hormone-releasing hormone nasal spray.

Answer: a. c. e. The child has enuresis during the day as well so a bedwetting alarm at night will not help. The child should avoid citrus fruits and high sugar foods that irritate the bladder. A behavioral modification chart is a good idea and a high fiber diet will help by preventing constipation.

96. A newborn has been diagnosed with bladder extrophy. What is the purpose of a suprapubic catheter?
    a. It is less painful than bladder catheterization.
    b. It does not require restraining the child like a bladder catheterization would.
    c. It is used to aspirate urine when the child hasn't voided for more than an hour.
    d. It is the only procedure that allows a small catheter to be used on a newborn.

Answer: c. It is used to aspirate urine when the child hasn't voided for more than an hour. It is actually more painful than a bladder catheterization and requires restraining the child.

97. The nurse checks the clients hourly output of urine as 70 cc/hour. What should the nurse do?
    a. Notify the physician immediately.
    b. Encourage the client to drink extra fluids.
    c. Tell the client to ambulate more.
    d. Recognize that this is a normal urine output.

Answer: d. 70 cc/hour is a normal urine output for an adult.

98. What is the purpose of asking the client with pyelonephritis to drink 3000 cc of fluids per day?
   a. To prevent urinary reflux.
   b. To prevent stasis of urine
   c. To decrease urine output
   d. To decrease residual urine

Answer: b. Drinking fluid will allow more urine to flow through the kidneys so that the bacteria can be flushed out.

99. The nurse is teaching the client about what foods to avoid if the client has calcium oxalate calculi?
   a. Celery
   b. Salmon
   c. Beets
   d. Bacon
   e. Whole wheat bread
   f. Asparagus

Answer: a. c. f. The goal is to reduce oxalate in the diet. Celery, beets, and asparagus are all high in an oxalate diet.

NCLEX: Genitourinary Disorders

100. The nurse is teaching a client and family about kidney disease. What does she say?
   a. It takes involvement of 90 percent of nephrons to have acute renal failure.
   b. There is a direct correlation between the amount of urine produced and the severity of kidney disease.
   c. Acute renal failure can happen in the presence of prolonged hypotension.
   d. The best test for kidney failure is the BUN level.

Answer: c. Acute renal failure can happen if there is prolonged hypotension. It takes 95 percent of nephrons to have acute renal failure. There is no correlation between the amount of urine produced and the degree of kidney disease. A better test for kidney failure is the creatinine level.

101. The nurse is giving a medication to a client with recurrent urinary tract infections. What medication is given?
   a. Levsin
   b. Urecholine
   c. Bactrim DS
   d. Pyridium

Answer: c. Bactrim DS is an antibiotic used to treat recurrent urinary tract infections. Pyridium is used to control the pain of urinary tract infections. Levsin is used for spastic bladder and urecholine is used to treat urinary retention.

102. A client is suffering from renal colic due to a ureteral stone. What is a priority nursing intervention?
a. Straining the urine
b. Giving morphine sulfate
c. Monitoring intake and output
d. Encourage ambulation

Answer: b. Giving a pain medication for renal colic is a priority intervention, while straining the urine and encouraging ambulation are secondary interventions. Monitoring intake and output is not necessary.

103. The nurse suspects kidney trauma after an automobile accident. What is a priority that the nurse should report?
a. Lethargy
b. Hypertension
c. Hematuria
d. Bradycardia

Answer: c. Hematuria is an important finding in suspected renal trauma and should be reported to the physician.

104. The nurse is caring for a client in acute renal failure. What is the clinical finding that the nurse should monitor as a priority?
a. Infection
b. Pain
c. Oliguria
d. Anemia

Answer: a. Infection is a big problem in acute renal failure and carries a high mortality rate. Pain is not seen in ARF and anemia is seen in CRF. Oliguria is a concern but is less of a problem than infection.

105. The client has acute renal failure. What lab report indicates the client is uremic?
a. BUN of 32 mg/dL
b. Serum calcium of 10.5 mg/d:
c. Serum potassium of 2.8 mg/dL
d. Urine specific gravity of 1.030

Answer: a. The client is said to be uremic if the BUN is elevated. A BUN of 32 mg/dL is too high and indicates uremia.

Conclusion

I hope you received a ton of value from this book. Remember, practice makes perfect so you will have to repeat these readings.

If you enjoyed this book, would you be kind enough to leave a review on Amazon? Your positive review can help others to see what kinds of helpful resources are out there!

Thank you and good luck on your medical endeavors!

- Chase Hassen

Nurse Superhero

Highly Recommended Books for Success

1. NCLEX: Cardiovascular System : 105 Nursing Practice and Rationales to Easily Crush the NCLEX!

2. NCLEX: Emergency Nursing : 105 Practice Questions and Rationales to Easily Crush the NCLEX!

3. Lab Values: 137 Values You Know to Easily Pass The NCLEX!

4. EKG Interpretation: 24 Hours or Less to Easily Pass the ECG Portion of the NCLEX!

5. Fluid and Electrolytes: 24 Hours or Less to Absolutely Crush the NCLEX Exam!

6. Nursing Careers: Easily Choose What Nursing Career Will Make Your 12 Hour Shift a Blast!

7. Night Shift: 10 Survival Tips for Nurses to Get Through The Night!

8. <u>NCLEX: Endocrine System : 105 Nursing Practice Questions and Rationales to EASILY Crush the NCLEX!</u>

And ***MUCH MUCH MORE***! Visit my amazon author page to see more at http://amzn.to/1HCtfSy

Made in the USA
Las Vegas, NV
05 August 2022